The intent of the author is only to offer general information to help you in your quest for emotional and spiritual welfare. In the event you use any of the information in this book for yourself or others, the author and the publisher assume no responsibility for your actions.

INTRODUCTION

- NO GYM REQUIRED -

WANT A SUREFIRE <u>HOME</u> WORKOUT SOLUTION TO FLATTEN YOUR BELLY, TONE FROM HEAD TO TOE AND 2X YOUR STRENGTH WHILE LOSING POUNDS AND INCHES – IN 30 DAYS?

Well, look no further.

The **30-DAY Total Body Super Circuit Home Workout Plan** is a <u>NO Fluff</u> workout plan that is <u>**NOT**</u> found on the internet telling you to perform, "10 of this and 10 of that ".

It's a science and proven based fitness routine created by Doug Bennett, Top American Trainer for the last 29 years, who has helped thousands and thousands of women transform both their health and body.

Simply follow this day-by-day top training HOME workout plan to get great results - even if you've failed in the past.

This Total Body 30 Day *blueprint* will easily fit into your busy schedule while transforming your entire body FASTER than any Home Workout Plan you have ever seen or used.

Each Week builds upon the previous week. Each level, beginner or advanced, Is designed to help ignite your metabolism, burn all your unwanted fat, build sexy, tone muscle and give you all the amazing results you desire.

This Fast Acting Total Body Transformation plan is guaranteed to start working within just a week, not months. You will immediately start to feel it working after just a few workouts.

Image how good it will feel in just 30 days to slip into your favorite jeans, boost energy, feel body confident, love your flat belly, while others comment, **"You look amazing!"**

Get your copy of the **30-DAY Total Body Super Circuit Home Workout Plan** now. This is your chance to finally get your fastest solution to transform your total body and belly without paying thousands for a Top Trainer.

PLEASE NOTE: THIS BOOK IS FITNESS WORKOUT PLAN NOT A DIET!

The diet included is a BONUS to help you get the best results. You may add this plan to your current Gym Workout to double your results or get Gym Quality Results right at home. This workout is challenging and takes some work for results. This is not a 7 minute gadget plan.

Steps To Get The Best Results.

- Always consult with your medical professional before starting any exercise and/or diet program.

- Read Over the diet and prepare all the foods that are necessary to get started.

- Recommended for best results but not all needed: Purchase 4-5 sets of dumbbells ranging from 5lbs to 20 lbs, a fitness ball 55 to 60 cm, 10 to 20 lb. medicine ball, fitness mat, running or walking shoes, jump rope and a blue or red fitness band.

- Challenge yourself with heavier weights.

- Eliminate access salts, sugars, refined carbohydrates, processed foods, artificial ingredients and alcohol for the 42 days.

- Try to maintain your amazing results with a healthy lifestyle. i.e. Daily exercise and a Mediterranean Diet.

Are You Ready To Get Going?

Let's Go! You can do this?

All the exercises have a picture to show the exact steps for the proper form. Exercise descriptions will tell you how to perform each exercise plus tell you what to do and not to do.

PLEASE READ BEFORE STARTING

The **30-DAY Total Body Super Circuit Home Workout Plan** and/or Doug Bennett, author, writes an exact diet and workout system that can help you get amazing total body changing results.

However, you must use it to get your desired results. Always, consult a qualified medical professional before starting this or any other diet and fitness program.

You are assuming all risk and liability by reading and using any of the material written in the The 30-DA Total Body Super Circuit Home Workout Plan and/or created by Douglas Bennett.

Always stop if you feel discomfort and seek medical help immediately. Results are based upon each individual. Results will vary. Thus, there is no guarantee based upon every individuals' certain limits, medical history, injuries or past fitness history.

All intellectual property created by Douglas Bennett including All material, protected by copyright, trademarks, service marks, diets, fitness programs, names, are owned, registered and/or licensed by the Body studio corp. all content in this book including but not limited to text, designs and content is collective work under the copyright laws and in the proprietary property of the Body studio corp. you agree not to print, modify, copy, broadcast, distribute, sell or transmit any content written in the **30-DAY Total Body Super Circuit Home Workout Plan**

Table of Contents

YOUR 30 DAY FITNESS PLAN

YOUR 30 DAY TOTAL BODY TONE UP PLAN

KEY POINTS FOR SUCCESS & IMPLEMENTATION

WARNING:

Always, consult with your medical professional before starting this exercise or any exercise program. These workouts are for informational purposes only and NOT a personal prescription. Please, perform at your own risk.

HOW TO GET THE BEST RESULTS (TIPS):

- Please give each exercise your best effort.
- **Cardio:** train with intensity.
- **Weights:** keep good form and challenge yourself with heavier weights. You will not get bulky with lifting heavier weights with good form If you're running, power walking and on a lean daily diet: 3-4 lean proteins (4-6 oz), 3-5 fresh veggies, steamed (1/2 – 1 cup), 1-2 complex carbs (1/4-1/2 cup), 1-2 fruit (1/4-1/2 cup) and lots of water.
- **Advanced:** You should be struggling towards the end of each set with the weight. If the weight is not challenging then increase.
- **Beginners:** should use light weights but keep good form by going down slower (2-4 seconds then powering up. Also, squeeze the muscle you're working !).
- Perform each circuit before moving onto next circuit.
- If you're very limited on time, just do 3 sets (3x) of each.
- Each circuit perform top to bottom and repeat as written.

HOW TO USE EACH DAYS WORKOUT (EXAMPLE):

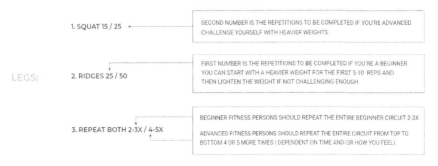

LEGS:

1. SQUAT 15 / 25 ← SECOND NUMBER IS THE REPETITIONS TO BE COMPLETED IF YOU'RE ADVANCED. CHALLENGE YOURSELF WITH HEAVIER WEIGHTS.

2. RIDGES 25 / 50 — FIRST NUMBER IS THE REPETITIONS TO BE COMPLETED IF YOU'RE A BEGINNER. YOU CAN START WITH A HEAVIER WEIGHT FOR THE FIRST 5-10 REPS AND THEN LIGHTEN THE WEIGHT IF NOT CHALLENGING ENOUGH.

3. REPEAT BOTH 2-3X / 4-5X — BEGINNER FITNESS PERSONS SHOULD REPEAT THE ENTIRE BEGINNER CIRCUIT 2-3X. ADVANCED FITNESS PERSONS SHOULD REPEAT THE ENTIRE CIRCUIT FROM TOP TO BOTTOM 4 OR 5 MORE TIMES (DEPENDENT ON TIME AND/OR HOW YOU FEEL).

30 DAY TOTAL BODY
FITNESS PLAN

 Day 1

LEGS:

1. AIR SQUAT 25/50

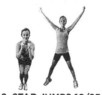

2. STAR JUMPS 10/25

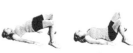

3. BRIDGES 25/50

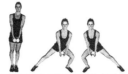

4. SIDE LUNGES 10 EACH LEG / 15 EACH LEG

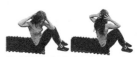

5. SIT UPS 10-20 / 30 - 50

REPEAT 2-4 X / 4-6 X OR AS MANY TIMES AS POSSIBLE IN 20 MINUTES
POWER UP BY ADDING: JOG OR POWER WALK 20-45 MINUTES

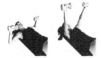 **Day 2**

ARMS:

1. FLAT PRESS, DBS 10/12 2. TRICEP BENCH 10/30 3. HAMMER CURLS 5-10 / 20-30

4. CURLS 15 / 20

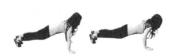

5. PUSH UPS, KNEES 10 / 25

REPEAT 2-4 X / 4-6 X OR AS MANY TIMES AS POSSIBLE IN 15-20 MINUTES
POWER UP BY ADDING: 1. HILL SPRINTS OR POWER WALK UP HILL 5 – 10X
2. PLUS POWER WALK OR JOG 15-30 MINUTES

12

30 DAY TOTAL BODY
FITNESS PLAN

 Day 3

ABS:

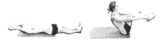

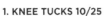

1. KNEE TUCKS 10/25   2. SIT UPS 10/25   3. BICYCLE 30 SEC / 1 MIN

     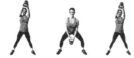

4. PLANK 30 SEC / 1 MIN   5. KETTLE BELL SWING 30 SEC / 1 MIN

REPEAT 2-4 X / 4-6 X OR AS MANY TIMES AS POSSIBLE IN 15-20 MINUTES
POWER UP BY ADDING: MOUNTAIN CLIMBERS > HIGH KNEE RUNNING > JUMPING JACKS
> SKATING > STAR JUMPS > CRUNCHES
BEGINNERS PERFORM EACH EXERCISE ABOVE 30 SEC AND REPEAT ALL 3-4X
WITHOUT REST AT OWN RISk.
ADVANCED PERFORM EACH EXERCISE ABOVE 1 MINUTE AND REPEAT ALL 3-4X
WITH NO REST AT OWN RISK.

 Day 4

LEGS:

     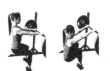   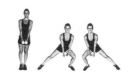

1. AIR SQUAT 25/50   2. SISSY SQUAT 25/50   3. LUNGES 10 EACH LEG / 20 EACH LEG

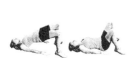   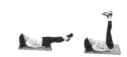

4. BRIDGES 25/50   5. PLIE SQUATS 25/50   6. LEG LIFTS TO HOP (ABS) 10/20

REPEAT 2-4 X / 4-6 X OR AS MANY TIMES AS POSSIBLE IN 15-20 MINUTES
POWER UP BY ADDING: JOG OR POWER WALK 20-45 MINUTES

30 DAY TOTAL BODY
FITNESS PLAN

 Day 5

ARMS:

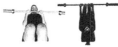 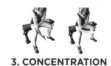

1. TRICEP CLOSE GRIP PRESS (BAR) 10/15 **2. TRICEP KICK BACKS 10 / 15-20** **3. CONCENTRATION CURLS 10 / 15 EACH ARM** **4. HAMMER CURLS 10 / 20**

5. SHOULDER PRESS 8-10 / 10-12 **6. SIDE RAISES 8-10 / 10-15** **7. NO BAR? TRICEP PUSH BACKS 15/25**

REPEAT 2-4 X / 4-6 X OR AS MANY TIMES AS POSSIBLE IN 15-20 MINUTES

POWER UP BY ADDING: 1. PUSH UPS 5-10 THEN JUMP UP AND SPRINT 30 YARDS, TURN DROP DOWN AND REPEAT 5- 10X   2. PLUS POWER WALK OR JOG 15-30 MINUTES

 Day 6

BUM:

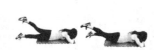

1. JUMPING SQUAT WITH MEDICINE BALL (10-20LB) 10/20 **2. SWIMMING 30 SEC / 1 MIN** **3. ONE LEG BRIDGES 25 EACH LEG / 50 EACH LEG**

 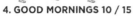 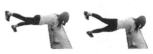

4. GOOD MORNINGS 10 / 15 **5. PLANK AND WALK FEET 10 / 30 EACH LEG**

REPEAT 2-4 X / 4-6 X OR AS MANY TIMES AS POSSIBLE IN 15 - 20 MINUTES

POWER UP BY ADDING: 1. WALK TREADMILL OR HILLS, 15 MINUTES, INCLINE 5-10 * (MEDICAL DEPENDENT AT OWN RISK)
2. JOB OR WALK STAIR STEPPER OR STEPS BLEACHERS (STAIRS) 2-3 MINUTES, REST 1 MINUTE AND REPEAT 3-4X

30 DAY TOTAL BODY
FITNESS PLAN

                                          ARMS:

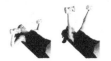 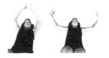

| 1. FLAT PRESS, | 2. FLAT FLIES | 3. HAMMER CURLS | 4. CURLS |
| DBS 10/12 | 10/15 | 5-10 / 20-30 | 15 / 20 |

 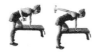

5. TRICEP BENCH   6. TRICEP KICK BACKS   7. SHOULDER PRESS
   10 / 30   10-12 / 12-15 EACH ARM   8-10 / 10-15

REPEAT 2-4 X / 4-6 X OR AS MANY TIMES AS POSSIBLE IN 15-20 MINUTES
POWER UP BY ADDING: CARDIO 30 – 60 MINUTES

Day 8   LEGS:

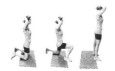

1. STAND UPS 10 / 25   2. STAR JUMPS   3. GLOBET SQUATS
      EACH LEG   10 / 25   25 / 50

4. JOG 100 YARDS TURN AND SPRINT BACK OR   5. JUMP ROPE OR JUMPING
   TREADMILL JOG 2 MIN, SPRINT 1 MIN   JACKS 30 SEC / 1MIN

REPEAT 2-4 X / 4-6 X OR AS MANY TIMES AS POSSIBLE IN 15-20 MINUTES
POWER UP BY ADDING: JOG OR POWER WALK 20-45 MINUTES

30 DAY TOTAL BODY
FITNESS PLAN

Day 9

ARMS, ABS:

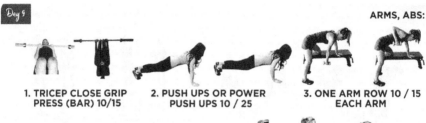

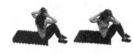

1. TRICEP CLOSE GRIP PRESS (BAR) 10/15

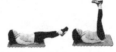

2. PUSH UPS OR POWER PUSH UPS 10 / 25

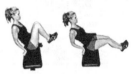

3. ONE ARM ROW 10 / 15 EACH ARM

4. SIT UPS WITH TWIST AT TOP 10-15 / 25-50

5. LEG RAISES TO A HOP 10 / 25

6. BENCH ACCORDIAN CRUNCH 10 / 25-50

REPEAT 2-4 X / 4-6 X OR AS MANY TIMES AS POSSIBLE IN 15-20 MINUTES

POWER UP BY ADDING: 1. STRAIGHT PUNCHES (HEAVY BAG OR WITH 2LB. DUMBBELLS, BOXING) 20 FOLLOWED BY 10 JUMPING JACKS AND REPEAT BOTH FOR 3 MINUTES, NO REST.
2. JOG 5-10 MINUTES   REPEAT BOTH ABOVE 1-3 X

Day 10

ARMS, SHOULDERS:

1. CURLS 10/15

2. HAMMER CURLS 10 / 25

3. SHOULDER PRESS 10 / 15

4. BENT OVER RAISES 10 / 12-15

5. SIDE RAISES 10 / 10-15

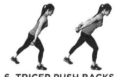

6. TRICEP PUSH BACKS 20 / 30

REPEAT 2-4 X / 4-6 X OR AS MANY TIMES AS POSSIBLE IN 15-20 MINUTES

POWER UP BY ADDING: MOUNTAIN CLIMBERS > HIGH KNEE RUNNING
> BURPEES > SKATING > STAR JUMPS > CRUNCHES
BEGINNERS PERFORM EACH EXERCISE ABOVE 30 SEC AND REPEAT ALL 3-4X WITHOUT REST AT OWN RISk.
ADVANCED PERFORM EACH EXERCISE ABOVE 1 MINUTE AND REPEAT ALL 3-4X WITH NO REST AT OWN RISk.

30 DAY TOTAL BODY
FITNESS PLAN

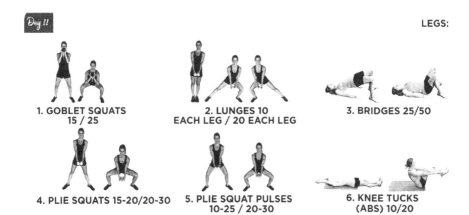

Day 11

LEGS:

1. GOBLET SQUATS
15 / 25

2. LUNGES 10
EACH LEG / 20 EACH LEG

3. BRIDGES 25/50

4. PLIE SQUATS 15-20/20-30

5. PLIE SQUAT PULSES
10-25 / 20-30

6. KNEE TUCKS
(ABS) 10/20

REPEAT 2-4 X / 4-6 X OR AS MANY TIMES AS POSSIBLE IN 15-20 MINUTES
POWER UP BY ADDING: JOG OR POWER WALK 20-45 MINUTES

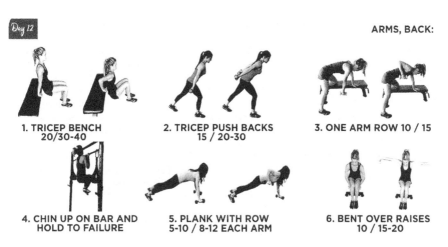

Day 12

ARMS, BACK:

1. TRICEP BENCH
20/30-40

2. TRICEP PUSH BACKS
15 / 20-30

3. ONE ARM ROW 10 / 15

4. CHIN UP ON BAR AND
HOLD TO FAILURE

5. PLANK WITH ROW
5-10 / 8-12 EACH ARM

6. BENT OVER RAISES
10 / 15-20

REPEAT 2-4 X / 4-6 X OR AS MANY TIMES AS POSSIBLE IN 15-20 MINUTES
POWER UP BY ADDING: CARDIO 30 - 60 MINUTES

30 DAY TOTAL BODY
FITNESS PLAN

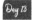

BUM:

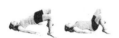

**1. BRIDGES 15 / 25
BOTH USE HEAVY WEIGHT**

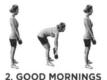

**2. GOOD MORNINGS
10 / 15**

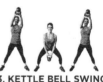

**3. KETTLE BELL SWING
30 SEC / 1 MINUTE**

**4. JUMPING SQUAT WITH
MEDICINE BALL 15 / 25**

**5. SKATING
1 MINUTE / 2 MINUTE**

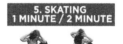

**6. SIT UPS WITH
TWIST 25 / 50**

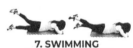

**7. SWIMMING
30 SEC / 1 MINUTE**

REPEAT 2-4 X / 4-6 X OR AS MANY TIMES AS POSSIBLE IN 15-20 MINUTES
POWER UP BY ADDING: 1. WALK TREADMILL OR HILLS, 15 MINUTES, INCLINE 5-10 *
(MEDICAL DEPENDENT AT OWN RISK)
2. JOB OR WALK STAIR STEPPER OR STEPS (BLEACHES) 2-3 MINUTES,
REST 1 MINUTE AND REPEAT 3-4X.

ABS:

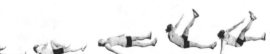

**1. BICYCLE
1 MINUTE / 2 MINUTES**

**2. X-OVERS ABS 10 / 25
EACH SIDE**

**3. HANGING KNEE
TUCKS 10 -15 / 15-25**

**4. PLANK ON FITNESS
BALL 30 SEC / 1 MINUTE**

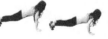

**5. PUSH UPS
10-15 / 25 - 50**

**6. SIT UPS WITH
TWIST 10 / 25**

**7. JUMP ROPE
1 MINUTE**

REPEAT 2-4 X / 4-6 X OR AS MANY TIMES AS POSSIBLE IN 15-20 MINUTES
POWER UP BY ADDING: 30 - 60 MINUTES OF CARDIO
(BIKE, SWIMMING, SPINNING, JOGGING, BOXING, ETC..)

30 DAY TOTAL BODY
FITNESS PLAN

 Day 15   **LEGS:**

   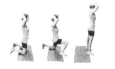

1. SQUAT 15 / 20   **2. SISSY SQUAT**   **2. STAND UPS 10 / *20**   **3. STAR JUMPS**
                       15 / 20   *(HOLD DUMBBELL UNDER CHIN, HORIZONTAL)   **10 / 25**
                                           EACH LEG

   JOG 100 YARDS TURN AND SPRINT BACK
                       OR TREADMILL JOG 2 MIN, SPRINT 1 MIN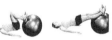

4. SIDE LUNGES   **6. FITNESS BALL BACK**
10 / 20 EACH LEG   **LEG CURLS 15 / 20**

REPEAT 2-4 X / 4-6 X OR AS MANY TIMES AS POSSIBLE IN 15-20 MINUTES

POWER UP BY ADDING: 1. JUMP ROPE 3-5 MINUTES
2. TRACK: SPRINTS 5 X 25 YARDS, 5 X 50 YARDS, 2 X 100 YARDS
    NOTE: BEGINNER SHOULD SPRINT AT 70% MAX, STRETCH AND
          PERFORM ONLY 2 OF EACH ABOVE.
3. TRACK: (ADVANCED ONLY) JOG ½ LAP, SPRINT ½ LAT, WALK ½ LAP AND REPEAT 2-3X.

Day 16   **ARMS, ABS:**

 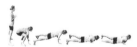

1. TRICEP CLOSE GRIP   **2. TRICEP BENCH**   **3. BURPEES 10 / 20**
PRESS (BAR) 10/15   **15 / 25-40**

 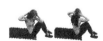

4. ONE ARM ROW   **5. SIT UPS WITH TWIST**   **6. TRICEP PUSH**   **7. LEG RAISES TO**
10 / 15 EACH ARM   **AT TOP 10-15 / 25-50**   **UPS 10 / 25**   **A HOP 10 / 25**

REPEAT 2-4 X / 4-6 X OR AS MANY TIMES AS POSSIBLE IN 15-20 MINUTES
POWER UP BY ADDING: 1. STRAIGHT BAG PUNCHES 20 FOLLOWED BY 10 JUMPING JACKS
                        AND REPEAT BOTH FOR 3 MINUTES, NO REST.
2. JUMP ROPE 1 MINUTE 3. PUSH UPS ON KNEES 10-15 / 20-30 REPEAT ALL ABOVE 4-6 X

30 DAY TOTAL BODY
FITNESS PLAN

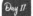 **Day 17**

ARMS, SHOULDERS:

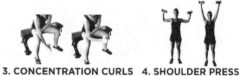

1. CURLS 10/15	2. HAMMER CURLS	3. CONCENTRATION CURLS	4. SHOULDER PRESS
	10 / 25	8 / 10-15 EACH ARM	10 / 15

5. SIDE RAISES	6. FRONT RAISES	7. HANGING KNEE TUCKS
10 / 10-15	8 / 10-12 EACH ARM	(ABS) 10-15 / 20-40

REPEAT 2-4 X / 4-6 X OR AS MANY TIMES AS POSSIBLE IN 15-20 MINUTES

POWER UP BY ADDING: MOUNTAIN CLIMBERS > HIGH KNEE RUNNING > BURPEES > SKATING > STAR JUMPS > CRUNCHES
BEGINNERS PERFORM EACH EXERCISE ABOVE 30 SEC AND REPEAT ALL 3-4X WITHOUT REST AT OWN RISK.
ADVANCED PERFORM EACH EXERCISE ABOVE 1 MINUTE AND REPEAT ALL 3-4X WITH NO REST AT OWN RISK.

 Day 18

BUM:

 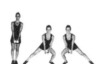

1. SQUAT W WEIGHT	2. LUNGES 10 EACH	3. SKATING	4. PLIE SQUATS
15 / 25	LEG / 20 EACH LEG	30 SECONDS / 1 MINUTE	15-20/20-30

5. PLIE SQUAT PULSES	6. KNEE TUCKS	7. 1-LEG STIFF LEG
10-25 / 20-30	10-15/20-30	DEAD LIFTS 10 / 15

REPEAT 2-4 X / 4-6 X OR AS MANY TIMES AS POSSIBLE IN 15-20 MINUTES

POWER UP BY ADDING: JOG OR POWER WALK 20-45 MINUTES

30 DAY TOTAL BODY
FITNESS PLAN

 Day 19

ARMS, BACK:

1. TRICEP PUSH BACKS
15 / 20-30

2. TRICEP KICK BACKS
15 / 15-20 EACH ARM
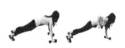

3. ONE ARM ROW
10 / 15
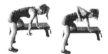

4. CHIN UP ON BAR AND
HOLD TO FAILURE

5. PLANK WITH ROW
5-10 / 8-12 EACH ARM

6. BENT OVER RAISES
10 /10-15

REPEAT 2-4 X / 4-6 X OR AS MANY TIMES AS POSSIBLE IN 15-20 MINUTES
POWER UP BY ADDING: 1. PUSH UPS 5-20 THEN JUMP UP AND SPRINT 30 YARDS,
TURN DROP DOWN AND REPEAT 5- 10X   2. PLUS POWER WALK OR JOG 20-45 MINUTES

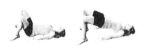 **Day 20**

BUM:

1. BRIDGES 15 / 25 * BOTH
USE HEAVY WEIGHT

2. GOOD MORNINGS
10 / 15
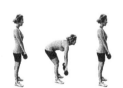

3. KETTLE BELL SWING
30 SEC / 1 MINUTE
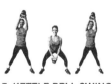

4. JUMPING SQUAT WITH
MEDICINE BALL 15 / 25

5. SWIMMING
1 MINUTE / 1 MINUTE
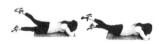

6. SIT UPS WITH TWIST
25 / 50
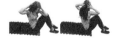

REPEAT 2-4 X / 4-6 X OR AS MANY TIMES AS POSSIBLE IN 15-20 MINUTES
POWER UP BY ADDING: 1. WALK TREADMILL OR HILLS, 15 MINUTES, INCLINE 5-10 *
(MEDICAL DEPENDENT AT OWN RISK)
2. JOB OR WALK STAIR STEPPER OR RUN STEPS (BLEACHES) 2-3 MINUTES,
   REST 1 MINUTE AND REPEAT 3-4X.
3. SPRINTS (ADVANCED ONLY) 3 X 300 METERS

30 DAY TOTAL BODY
FITNESS PLAN

 Day 21   **ABS:**

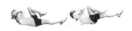

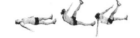

1. BICYCLE
1 MINUTE / 2 MINUTES

2. X-OVERS ABS
10 / 25 EACH SIDE

3. HANGING KNEE TUCKS
10 -15 / 15-25

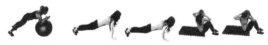

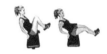

4. PLANK ON BALL
30 SEC / 1 MINUTE

5. PUSH UPS
10-15 / 25 - 50

6. SIT UPS
10 / 25

7. ACCORDIAN CRUNCHES,
BENCH 10-20 / 30-50

REPEAT 2-4 X / 4-6 X OR AS MANY TIMES AS POSSIBLE IN 15-20 MINUTES

POWER UP BY ADDING: 30 – 60 MINUTES OF CARDIO
(BIKE, SWIMMING, SPINNING, JOGGING, BOXING, ETC..)

Day 22   **LEGS:**

1. GOBLET SQUAT
15 / 20

2. AIR SQUAT
25 / 50

3. JUMP ROPE OR JUMPING
JACKS WITH FIST 1 MIN

4. STAR JUMPS
10 / 25

5. JUMP ROPE OR JUMPING
JACKS WITH FIST 1 MIN

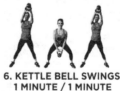

7. JOG 2 MINUTES, SPRINT
30 SECONDS – 1 MINUTE

6. KETTLE BELL SWINGS
1 MINUTE / 1 MINUTE

REPEAT 2-4 X / 4-6 X OR AS MANY TIMES AS POSSIBLE IN 15-20 MINUTES

POWER UP BY ADDING: 1. JOG 3-5 MINUTES
2. TRACK: SPRINTS 6 X 25 YARDS, 5 X 50 YARDS, 3 X 100 YARDS
   NOTE: BEGINNER SHOULD SPRINT AT 70% MAX,
      STRETCH AND PERFORM ONLY 2 OF EACH ABOVE.
3. TRACK: (ADVANCED ONLY) JOG ½ LAP, SPRINT ½ LAT, WALK ½ LAP AND REPEAT 2-4X.

30 DAY TOTAL BODY
FITNESS PLAN

 Day 23   ARMS:

  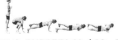

1. TRICEP CLOSE GRIP   2. BURPEES 10 / 20   3. ONE ARM ROW   4. CHIN UP ON BAR
PRESS (BAR) 10/15   10 / 15 EACH ARM AND HOLD TO FAILURE

                          6. KICK BACKS WITH BAND
                          20 PULSES / 30 PULSES EACH ARM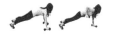

5. KICK BACKS   7. PLANK WITH ROW
10 / 15 EACH ARM   8-10 / 10-15 EACH ARM

REPEAT 2-4 X / 4-6 X OR AS MANY TIMES AS POSSIBLE IN 15-20 MINUTES
POWER UP BY ADDING: REPEAT 2-4 X / 4-6 X OR AS MANY TIMES AS POSSIBLE
IN 15-20 MINUTES.

4. STRAIGHT BAG PUNCHES 40 FOLLOWED BY 10 JUMPING JACKS
   AND REPEAT BOTH FOR 4 MINUTES, NO REST
5. JUMP ROPE 1 MINUTE   6. PUSH UPS ON KNEES 10-15 / 20-30 (REPEAT ALL ABOVE 4-6 X)

 Day 24   ARMS, SHOULDERS:

1. CURLS 15/20   2. HAMMER CURLS 10 / 25   3. CONCENTRATION CURLS
                                                        8 / 10-15 EACH ARM

4. SHOULDER PRESS 10 / 15   5. SIDE RAISES 10 / 10-15   6. FRONT RAISES
                                                               8 / 10-12 EACH ARM

REPEAT 2-4 X / 4-6 X OR AS MANY TIMES AS POSSIBLE IN 15-20 MINUTES

POWER UP BY ADDING: MOUNTAIN CLIMBERS > HIGH KNEE RUNNING >
                          BURPEES > SKATING > STAR JUMPS > CRUNCHES
BEGINNERS PERFORM EACH EXERCISE ABOVE 45 SEC AND REPEAT ALL 3-4X
WITHOUT REST AT OWN RISK.
ADVANCED PERFORM EACH EXERCISE ABOVE 1.5 MINUTES AND REPEAT ALL 3-4X
WITH NO REST AT OWN RISKS.

30 DAY TOTAL BODY
FITNESS PLAN

 Day 25   **LEGS:**

1. SQUAT W WEIGHT
15 / 25

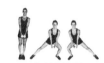

2. LUNGES
10 EACH LEG / 20 EACH LEG

3. SKATING
30 SECONDS / 2 MINUTE

4. PLIE SQUATS
15-20/20-30

5. PLIE SQUAT PULSES
10-25 / 20-30

6. STEP UPS ON BENCH
10 EACH LEG / 20 EACH LEG

REPEAT 2-4 X / 4-6 X OR AS MANY TIMES AS POSSIBLE IN 15-20 MINUTES
POWER UP BY ADDING: JOG OR POWER WALK 30-45 MINUTES

 Day 26   **ARMS, BACK:**

1. TRICEP BENCH
20 / *20-30 WITH WEIGHT

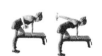

2. TRICEP KICK BACKS
15 / 15-20 EACH ARM

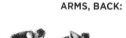

3. ONE ARM ROW 5 / 10 EACH
ARM, HEAVY FOR BOTH

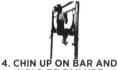

4. CHIN UP ON BAR AND
HOLD TO FAILURE

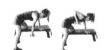

5. ONE ARM ROW 10 / 15
LIGHTER THAN #3 EACH ARM

6. BENT OVER
RAISES 10 /10-15

REPEAT 2-4 X / 4-6 X OR AS MANY TIMES AS POSSIBLE IN 15-20 MINUTES
POWER UP BY ADDING: 1. PUSH UPS 5-20 THEN JUMP UP AND SPRINT 30 YARDS,
TURN DROP DOWN AND REPEAT 5- 10X
2. POWER WALK, JOG OR BIKE 15-45 MINUTES

30 DAY TOTAL BODY
FITNESS PLAN

 Day 27

BUM:

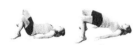

1. BRIDGES 15 / 25
BOTH USE HEAVY WEIGHT

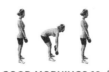

2. GOOD MORNINGS 10 / 15

3. KETTLE BELL SWING
30 SEC / 1 MINUTE

4. JUMPING SQUAT WITH
MEDICINE BALL 15 / 25

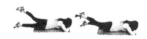

5. SWIMMING
1 MINUTE / 1 MINUTE

6. SIT UPS WITH
TWIST 25 / 50

REPEAT 2-4 X / 4-6 X OR AS MANY TIMES AS POSSIBLE IN 15-20 MINUTES
POWER UP BY ADDING: 1. WALK TREADMILL OR HILLS, 15 MINUTES, INCLINE 5-10
* (MEDICAL DEPENDENT AT OWN RISK)
2. JOB OR WALK STAIR STEPPER OR RUN STEPS (BLEACHES) 2-3 MINUTES,
REST 1 MINUTE AND REPEAT 3-4X
3. SPRINTS (ADVANCED ONLY) 3 X 300 METERS

 Day 28

ABS:

1. BICYCLE
1 MINUTE / 2 MINUTES

2. X-OVERS ABS 10 / 25
EACH SIDE

3. HANGING KNEE
TUCKS 10 -15 / 15-25

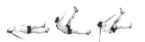

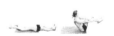

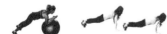

4. PLANK ON BALL   **5. PUSH UPS**   **6. SIT UPS 10 / 25** **7. ACCORDIAN CRUNCHES,**
30 SEC / 1 MINUTE   **10-15 / 25 - 50**   **BENCH 10-20 / 30-50**

REPEAT 2-4 X / 4-6 X OR AS MANY TIMES AS POSSIBLE IN 15-20 MINUTES
POWER UP BY ADDING: 30 – 60 MINUTES OF CARDIO (BIKE, SWIMMING, SPINNING
JOGGING, BOXING, ETC..)

30 DAY TOTAL BODY
FITNESS PLAN

 Day 29

JOG OR POWER WALK 45 – 90 MINUTES

 Day 30

CARDIO:

JOG OR POWER WALK 45 – 90 MINUTES

DIET

30 DAY KICK START DIET

(NOTE: NOT TO BE SHARED OR REPLICATED)

This is not a personal diet. It's a guide to kick your metabolism up a notch, lose pounds and help you get defined and tone muscles. Always consult your doctor before starting any diet plan!

- Eliminate ALL processed foods, chemicals, artificial sugars, hydrogenated fats and fatty meats. Eat only all natural foods. Increase lean protein. Consume little sugar and starch. For starches eat short grain brown rice, root veggies and wild rice. Fill up with organic veggies (frozen or fresh) and power greens (kale, spinach, mustard greens). Eating good fats will help you fill less hungry: fish oil, EVO, avocado, raw nuts or nut butters, organic butter, Earth Balance butter spread.

- Drink water at least 6x per day and take a daily WHOLE FOODS BASED MULTIPLE VITAMIN and electrolyte supplement.

- IF you are hungry then increase your fats by a tablespoon a day and/or complex carbs by 1-2 cups. Make sure to track your food using My fitness pal and/or the Fitness and Habit Tracker in this guide.

- On this diet, you will be hungry for the first few days as this is normal. Please consume greens whenever starving and/or a lean protein with a tsp good fat. You should never starve but being not full is good.

Daily Goal (Food Intake, servings):

Greens (3-5), Lean Protein (3-4),

Good Carbs (1), Good Fats (2),

TRY TO PERFORM CARDIO OR WORKOUT BEFORE MEAL 2

MEAL 1

Black Coffee or Green Tea Lemon and Fresh Water

1 cup of watermelon or blackberries, blueberries and or strawberries

*ABSOLUTELY NO BANANAS

MEAL 2

(9-11 am)

Protein + Fat + Veggie Optional : choose 1 below

- ½ cup of fruit (blackberries, blueberries, strawberries) and hardboiled egg
- Organic chicken sausage 1-2 link or patty, 1 egg white, tsp EARTH BALANCE BUTTER
- Tofu scramble with 1 tbsp avocado
- 3 slices natural turkey bacon, 1 EGG WHITE, tsp EARTH BALANCE
- ½ cup Low-Fat Cottage cheese, ¼ cup blueberries, 1-ounce raw nuts
- Protein Drink: spring water, 2 scoops
- 3 egg whites, Dragon Hot Sauce found at Trader Joes, 1 tbsp avocado
- ORGAIN PROTEIN POWDER, 2 SCOOPS ALL GREENS, 1/4 cup unsweetened almond milk, 1 tbsp avocado
- 1/2 cup fresh fruit, 2 tbsp. wheat germ and ½ cup natural, Greek or Non-dairy yogurt (unsweetened).
- 2 egg whites, organic turkey bacon (2-3 slices), 1 ounce nuts
- 3-4 slices all natural deli turkey or chicken wrapped in lettuce with shredded beets, carrots and 1 tsp avocado

No time to make food in the morning? Eat a prepared HARD BOILED EGG, 1 OUNCE RAW ALMONDS

MEAL 3

PROTEIN + SALAD + VEGGIE + LOW CARB: choose 1 below or make your own meal

- 1 CUP Arugula or Kale Salad with ½ cup veggies, 3-4 oz protein (Tofu, Tempeh, Beans, Tuna in water, Chicken or Turkey (deli or grilled), shrimp, Fish, Ground Meat)
- 3-4 ounces organic deli meat, wrapped in Boston Lettuce and Filled with Veggies
- Coconut water, protein bar (ONE or Good Bar), 2 oz raw nuts
- slice eziekeil toast with veggies, slice cheese, 2 oz protein and salad
- stir fry 3-4 oz fish, tofu or shrimp, 1 cup sautéed veggies (cook in broth), 1 handful dried cranberries or golgi berries, 1 ounce seed and or nuts
- 4 ounces ground turkey or chicken mixed with ½ cup brown rice, 1 cup veggies and topped with favorite dressing (organic bbq, hot sauce, RAOs marinara, just to name a few)
- 1 cup Ezekiel Almond Cereal with 1 cup nondairy, unsweetened
- beverage (coconut or almond)
- 1-2 cups organic sautéed or steamed veggies with tsp. extra
- virgin olive oil and 3-4 ounces lean protein
- 3-4 slices organic deli chicken or turkey slices, low carb (engine 2 or Ezekiel wrap), greens, avocado (chopped tbsp), mustard or vinaigrette, sweet potato

- Slice Ezekiel toast or Boston lettuce wrap, 3 oz tuna (whole foods: POLL LINE BRAND or trader joes), veggies,

- VEGAN CEREAL: mix ½ cup hemp hearts, 1 ounce goji berries, 1 tbsp flax seeds, 1 ounce slithered raw almonds. Top with non-dairy beverage

- 1-2 CUPS Favorite Natural broth, low-fat soup (many varieties found at whole foods in natural food section).

- Cauliflower crust (found frozen section Trader Joes or Whole foods), topped with veggies and 3 0z of protein of choice, tsp fat and 3-4 oz protein

Example: arugula, chopped tomato, ½ oz feta, basil, 2-3 oz ground or chopped grilled chicken and balsamic vinegar.

MAKE YOUR OWN MEAL 3 with veggies, greens and protein:

CHOOSE AS BELOW (GREENS, VEGGIES, PROTEIN)

*Greens (1-3 Cups choices below): Romaine Lettuce

Baby Kale

Baby Spinach and Red Spinach Arugula

Red and Green Leaf Lettuce

Dandelion

Swiss Chard

*Veggies (1/2 -2 cups choices below):

Broccoli

Red Onions

Kale

Spinach

Peppers

Asparagus

Tomatoes (fruit)

Asparagus

Edamame

Cabbage

Cauliflower

Celery

Turnips

Zucchini

Cucumber

*CARBS (1/2 cup choices below):

Sweet potato

quinoa

wheat berry

red bliss potato brown

rice (short grain best), wild rice or jasmine rice

Protein (3-6 ounces choices below):

- Light Tuna (in water (wild caught, all natural with no
- preservatives)
- Fish (wild salmon, shrimp, white fish, scallops)
- Grass Fed, Organic: Chicken Breast, Ground Chicken & Turkey
- 93% lean, Turkey,
- Grass Fed, Organic: Beef (top round, sirloin, flank), Ground
- Beef 93% lean
- Tempeh, Tofu
- Egg Whites
- Lentils (1/4 cup)

MEAL 4: SNACK (OPTIONAL)

- Protein (choose 1)

- 2 scoops protein powder, ice and water

- Turkey jerky

- 2 ounces raw nuts

- Hard boiled egg

- ½ cup unsweetened LOW-FAT Greek or Non-Dairy Yogurt with 1 tbsp Hemp seeds,

DON'T WANT TO EAT? YOU DON'T HAVE TOO. DRINK LEMON AND WATER OR COCONUT WATER ORIGINAL.

MEAL 5:

Clean Dinner Suggestions (fewer the ingredients the better): 3-6 ounces protein + 1 cup veggies and or greens (NO CARB UNLESS VEGETERIAN)

- Ground lean Protein (organic beef -1 x week only, chicken or turkey) mixed with sautéed veggies 1-3 cups.

- 3-6 ounces White Fish baked in tinfoil with lemon juice, white wine and black pepper. Served with greens and stir fried veggies.

- 3-5 ounces Grilled Free Range Chicken sliced and placed on greens with veggies and Newman's Own Lite Caesar Dressing.

- ½ cup Ground Protein (organic beef, chicken or turkey) mixed with ¼ cup fresh pico de gallo over 3 cups lettuce and pinch or natural Mexican shredded cheese (Cabot).

- 4-6 ounces Grilled Wild Salmon topped with chopped cucumber, tomato and lemon juice. Serve with wedge of Pink Grapefruit and salad.

- Scrambled Egg Whites with light cheese and turkey bacon. Two slices tomato and salad with veggies.

- 4-6 ounces Grilled Chicken topped with Bruschetta. Served with steamed asparagus and spinach.

- Organic Bone Broth Chicken Soup with veggies. Served with salad.

- Organic Veggie Broth Soup. Served with quinoa, raw nuts and lentils.

- Tofu sautéed in coconut oil with sliced carrots, chopped onion, garlic clove, cubed sweet potato and seasoning (curry, sea salt and cumin). Served with quinoa OR brown rice, raw nuts and lentils.

- Veggie Chili (lentils, white beans) in a tomato broth with sautéed carrots, onions and peppers. Add tofu or organic ground protein.

  Late Night Snack (select one only if needed)

- 2 ounces deli slices

- protein drink 2 scoops powder with 8 ounces unsweetened almond milk (Casein or Orgain Organic Protein Powder)

  ½ cup low-fat cottage cheese.

DRINK DAILY: Herbal Teas, 1-gallon water a day with or without lemon, green tea and black coffee.

YOUR FITNESS
&
HABITS TRACKER

Dietary Journal

DAY 1

DIETARY	Vegetable	Protein	Carbohydrate	Fat	Dairy	Fruit	Calories
Breakfast							
Snack							
Lunch							
Snack							
Dinner							
Daily Food Totals							

DID YOU REACH YOUR DAILY DIETARY GOAL?   YES   NO   *IF NO, why?*   TIME   WORK   STRESS   HUNGRY   MOOD

DID YOU TAKE YOURMULTIPLE VITAMIN?   YES   NO   OTHER SUPPLEMENTS ....

EAT OUT?   YES   NO   IF YES, GOOD OR BAD   CURRENT WEIGHT .... POUNDS.

WATER INTAKE (CHECK OFF)   8 OUNCES

EXTRA COMMENTS:
....

Dietary Journal

DIETARY	Vegetable	Protein	Carbohydrate	Fat	Dairy	Fruit	Calories
Breakfast							
Snack							
Lunch							
Snack							
Dinner							
Daily Food Totals							

DID YOU REACH YOUR DAILY DIETARY GOAL?   YES   NO   *IF NO, why?*   TIME   WORK   STRESS   HUNGRY   MOOD

DID YOU TAKE YOUR MULTIPLE VITAMIN?   YES   NO   OTHER SUPPLEMENTS ....

EAT OUT?   YES   NO   IF YES, GOOD OR BAD   CURRENT WEIGHT .... POUNDS.

WATER INTAKE (CHECK OFF)   8 OUNCES

EXTRA COMMENTS:
....

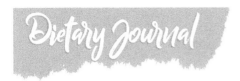

DAY 3

DIETARY	Vegetable	Protein	Carbohydrate	Fat	Dairy	Fruit	Calories
Breakfast							
Snack							
Lunch							
Snack							
Dinner							
Daily Food Totals							

DID YOU REACH YOUR DAILY DIETARY GOAL? YES NO *IF NO, why?* TIME WORK STRESS HUNGRY MOOD

DID YOU TAKE YOURMULTIPLE VITAMIN? YES NO OTHER SUPPLEMENTS ....

EAT OUT? YES NO IF YES, GOOD OR BAD CURRENT WEIGHT .... POUNDS.

WATER INTAKE (CHECK OFF) 8 OUNCES

EXTRA COMMENTS:
....

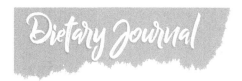

DAY 4

DIETARY	Vegetable	Protein	Carbohydrate	Fat	Dairy	Fruit	Calories
Breakfast							
Snack							
Lunch							
Snack							
Dinner							
Daily Food Totals							

DID YOU REACH YOUR DAILY DIETARY GOAL?　　YES　　　NO　*IF NO, why?*　　TIME　　WORK　　STRESS　　HUNGRY　　MOOD

DID YOU TAKE YOUR MULTIPLE VITAMIN?　　YES　　　NO　　OTHER SUPPLEMENTS ....

EAT OUT?　　YES　　NO　　IF YES, GOOD OR BAD　　CURRENT WEIGHT .... POUNDS.

WATER INTAKE (CHECK OFF)　　　　　　　8 OUNCES

EXTRA COMMENTS:
....

Dietary Journal

DAY 5

DIETARY	Vegetable	Protein	Carbohydrate	Fat	Dairy	Fruit	Calories
Breakfast							
Snack							
Lunch							
Snack							
Dinner							
Daily Food Totals							

DID YOU REACH YOUR DAILY DIETARY GOAL?   YES   NO   *IF NO, why?*   TIME   WORK   STRESS   HUNGRY   MOOD

DID YOU TAKE YOURMULTIPLE VITAMIN?   YES   NO   OTHER SUPPLEMENTS ....

EAT OUT?   YES   NO   IF YES, GOOD OR BAD   CURRENT WEIGHT .... POUNDS.

WATER INTAKE (CHECK OFF)   8 OUNCES

EXTRA COMMENTS:
....

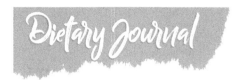

DIETARY	Vegetable	Protein	Carbohydrate	Fat	Dairy	Fruit	Calories
Breakfast							
Snack							
Lunch							
Snack							
Dinner							
Daily Food Totals							

DID YOU REACH YOUR DAILY DIETARY GOAL?   YES   NO *IF NO, why?*   TIME   WORK   STRESS   HUNGRY   MOOD

DID YOU TAKE YOUR MULTIPLE VITAMIN?   YES   NO   OTHER SUPPLEMENTS ....

EAT OUT?   YES   NO   IF YES, GOOD OR BAD   CURRENT WEIGHT .... POUNDS.

WATER INTAKE (CHECK OFF)   8 OUNCES

EXTRA COMMENTS:
....

Dietary Journal

DAY 7

DIETARY	Vegetable	Protein	Carbohydrate	Fat	Dairy	Fruit	Calories
Breakfast							
Snack							
Lunch							
Snack							
Dinner							
Daily Food Totals							

DID YOU REACH YOUR DAILY DIETARY GOAL?　　YES　　NO　　*IF NO, why?*　　TIME　　WORK　　STRESS　　HUNGRY　　MOOD

DID YOU TAKE YOUR MULTIPLE VITAMIN?　　YES　　NO　　OTHER SUPPLEMENTS ....

EAT OUT?　　YES　　NO　　IF YES, GOOD OR BAD　　CURRENT WEIGHT .... POUNDS.

WATER INTAKE (CHECK OFF)　　　　　　　　　8 OUNCES

EXTRA COMMENTS:
....

Dietary Journal

DIETARY	Vegetable	Protein	Carbohydrate	Fat	Dairy	Fruit	Calories
Breakfast							
Snack							
Lunch							
Snack							
Dinner							
Daily Food Totals							

DID YOU REACH YOUR DAILY DIETARY GOAL?   YES   NO   **IF NO, why?**   TIME   WORK   STRESS   HUNGRY   MOOD

DID YOU TAKE YOUR MULTIPLE VITAMIN?   YES   NO   OTHER SUPPLEMENTS ....

EAT OUT?   YES   NO   IF YES, GOOD OR BAD   CURRENT WEIGHT .... POUNDS.

WATER INTAKE (CHECK OFF)   8 OUNCES

EXTRA COMMENTS:
....

Dietary Journal

DIETARY	Vegetable	Protein	Carbohydrate	Fat	Dairy	Fruit	Calories
Breakfast							
Snack							
Lunch							
Snack							
Dinner							
Daily Food Totals							

DID YOU REACH YOUR DAILY DIETARY GOAL?   YES   NO   *IF NO, why?*   TIME   WORK   STRESS   HUNGRY   MOOD

DID YOU TAKE YOURMULTIPLE VITAMIN?   YES   NO   OTHER SUPPLEMENTS ....

EAT OUT?   YES   NO   IF YES, GOOD OR BAD   CURRENT WEIGHT .... POUNDS.

WATER INTAKE (CHECK OFF)   8 OUNCES

EXTRA COMMENTS:
....

Dietary Journal

DAY 10

DIETARY	Vegetable	Protein	Carbohydrate	Fat	Dairy	Fruit	Calories
Breakfast							
Snack							
Lunch							
Snack							
Dinner							
Daily Food Totals							

DID YOU REACH YOUR DAILY DIETARY GOAL?   YES   NO   *IF NO, why*?   TIME   WORK   STRESS   HUNGRY   MOOD

DID YOU TAKE YOURMULTIPLE VITAMIN?   YES   NO   OTHER SUPPLEMENTS ....

EAT OUT?   YES   NO   IF YES, GOOD OR BAD   CURRENT WEIGHT .... POUNDS.

WATER INTAKE (CHECK OFF)   8 OUNCES

EXTRA COMMENTS:
....

Dietary Journal

DAY 11

DIETARY	Vegetable	Protein	Carbohydrate	Fat	Dairy	Fruit	Calories
Breakfast							
Snack							
Lunch							
Snack							
Dinner							
Daily Food Totals							

DID YOU REACH YOUR DAILY DIETARY GOAL?   YES   NO   *IF NO, why?*   TIME   WORK   STRESS   HUNGRY   MOOD

DID YOU TAKE YOUR MULTIPLE VITAMIN?   YES   NO   OTHER SUPPLEMENTS ....

EAT OUT?   YES   NO   IF YES, GOOD OR BAD   CURRENT WEIGHT .... POUNDS.

WATER INTAKE (CHECK OFF)   8 OUNCES

EXTRA COMMENTS:
....

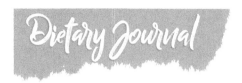

DAY 12

DIETARY	Vegetable	Protein	Carbohydrate	Fat	Dairy	Fruit	Calories
Breakfast							
Snack							
Lunch							
Snack							
Dinner							
Daily Food Totals							

DID YOU REACH YOUR DAILY DIETARY GOAL?   YES   NO *IF NO, why?*   TIME   WORK   STRESS   HUNGRY   MOOD

DID YOU TAKE YOURMULTIPLE VITAMIN?   YES   NO   OTHER SUPPLEMENTS ....

EAT OUT?   YES   NO   IF YES, GOOD OR BAD   CURRENT WEIGHT .... POUNDS.

WATER INTAKE (CHECK OFF)   8 OUNCES

EXTRA COMMENTS:
....

Dietary Journal

DAY 13

DIETARY	Vegetable	Protein	Carbohydrate	Fat	Dairy	Fruit	Calories
Breakfast							
Snack							
Lunch							
Snack							
Dinner							
Daily Food Totals							

DID YOU REACH YOUR DAILY DIETARY GOAL?   YES   NO *IF NO, why?*   TIME   WORK   STRESS   HUNGRY   MOOD

DID YOU TAKE YOURMULTIPLE VITAMIN?   YES   NO   OTHER SUPPLEMENTS ....

EAT OUT?   YES   NO   IF YES, GOOD OR BAD   CURRENT WEIGHT .... POUNDS.

WATER INTAKE (CHECK OFF)   8 OUNCES

EXTRA COMMENTS:
....

Dietary Journal

DAY 14

DIETARY	Vegetable	Protein	Carbohydrate	Fat	Dairy	Fruit	Calories
Breakfast							
Snack							
Lunch							
Snack							
Dinner							
Daily Food Totals							

DID YOU REACH YOUR DAILY DIETARY GOAL?   YES   NO   *IF NO, why?*   TIME   WORK   STRESS   HUNGRY   MOOD

DID YOU TAKE YOUR MULTIPLE VITAMIN?   YES   NO   OTHER SUPPLEMENTS ....

EAT OUT?   YES   NO   IF YES, GOOD OR BAD   CURRENT WEIGHT .... POUNDS.

WATER INTAKE (CHECK OFF)   8 OUNCES

EXTRA COMMENTS:
....

Dietary Journal

DIETARY	Vegetable	Protein	Carbohydrate	Fat	Dairy	Fruit	Calories
Breakfast							
Snack							
Lunch							
Snack							
Dinner							
Daily Food Totals							

DID YOU REACH YOUR DAILY DIETARY GOAL?   YES   NO   *IF NO, why?*   TIME   WORK   STRESS   HUNGRY   MOOD

DID YOU TAKE YOURMULTIPLE VITAMIN?   YES   NO   OTHER SUPPLEMENTS ....

EAT OUT?   YES   NO   IF YES, GOOD OR BAD   CURRENT WEIGHT .... POUNDS.

WATER INTAKE (CHECK OFF)   8 OUNCES

EXTRA COMMENTS:
....

Dietary Journal

DIETARY	Vegetable	Protein	Carbohydrate	Fat	Dairy	Fruit	Calories
Breakfast							
Snack							
Lunch							
Snack							
Dinner							
Daily Food Totals							

DID YOU REACH YOUR DAILY DIETARY GOAL?   YES   NO   *IF NO, why?*   TIME   WORK   STRESS   HUNGRY   MOOD

DID YOU TAKE YOUR MULTIPLE VITAMIN?   YES   NO   OTHER SUPPLEMENTS ....

EAT OUT?   YES   NO   IF YES, GOOD OR BAD   CURRENT WEIGHT .... POUNDS.

WATER INTAKE (CHECK OFF)   8 OUNCES

EXTRA COMMENTS:
....

Dietary Journal

DIETARY	Vegetable	Protein	Carbohydrate	Fat	Dairy	Fruit	Calories
Breakfast							
Snack							
Lunch							
Snack							
Dinner							
Daily Food Totals							

DID YOU REACH YOUR DAILY DIETARY GOAL?   YES   NO *IF NO, why?*   TIME   WORK   STRESS   HUNGRY   MOOD

DID YOU TAKE YOURMULTIPLE VITAMIN?   YES   NO   OTHER SUPPLEMENTS ....

EAT OUT?   YES   NO   IF YES, GOOD OR BAD   CURRENT WEIGHT .... POUNDS.

WATER INTAKE (CHECK OFF)   8 OUNCES

EXTRA COMMENTS:
....

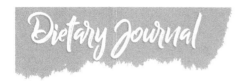

DIETARY	Vegetable	Protein	Carbohydrate	Fat	Dairy	Fruit	Calories
Breakfast							
Snack							
Lunch							
Snack							
Dinner							
Daily Food Totals							

DID YOU REACH YOUR DAILY DIETARY GOAL?   YES   NO   *IF NO, why?*   TIME   WORK   STRESS   HUNGRY   MOOD

DID YOU TAKE YOURMULTIPLE VITAMIN?   YES   NO   OTHER SUPPLEMENTS ....

EAT OUT?   YES   NO   IF YES, GOOD OR BAD   CURRENT WEIGHT .... POUNDS.

WATER INTAKE (CHECK OFF)   8 OUNCES

EXTRA COMMENTS:
....

Dietary Journal

DIETARY	Vegetable	Protein	Carbohydrate	Fat	Dairy	Fruit	Calories
Breakfast							
Snack							
Lunch							
Snack							
Dinner							
Daily Food Totals							

DID YOU REACH YOUR DAILY DIETARY GOAL?   YES   NO   *IF NO, why*?   TIME   WORK   STRESS   HUNGRY   MOOD

DID YOU TAKE YOURMULTIPLE VITAMIN?   YES   NO   OTHER SUPPLEMENTS ....

EAT OUT?   YES   NO   IF YES, GOOD OR BAD   CURRENT WEIGHT .... POUNDS.

WATER INTAKE (CHECK OFF)   8 OUNCES

EXTRA COMMENTS:
....

Dietary Journal

DIETARY	Vegetable	Protein	Carbohydrate	Fat	Dairy	Fruit	Calories
Breakfast							
Snack							
Lunch							
Snack							
Dinner							
Daily Food Totals							

DID YOU REACH YOUR DAILY DIETARY GOAL? YES NO **IF NO, why?** TIME WORK STRESS HUNGRY MOOD

DID YOU TAKE YOURMULTIPLE VITAMIN? YES NO OTHER SUPPLEMENTS ....

EAT OUT? YES NO IF YES, GOOD OR BAD CURRENT WEIGHT .... POUNDS.

WATER INTAKE (CHECK OFF) 8 OUNCES

EXTRA COMMENTS:
....

Dietary Journal

DAY 21

DIETARY	Vegetable	Protein	Carbohydrate	Fat	Dairy	Fruit	Calories
Breakfast							
Snack							
Lunch							
Snack							
Dinner							
Daily Food Totals							

DID YOU REACH YOUR DAILY DIETARY GOAL?   YES   NO   *IF NO, why?*   TIME   WORK   STRESS   HUNGRY   MOOD

DID YOU TAKE YOUR MULTIPLE VITAMIN?   YES   NO   OTHER SUPPLEMENTS ....

EAT OUT?   YES   NO   IF YES, GOOD OR BAD   CURRENT WEIGHT .... POUNDS.

WATER INTAKE (CHECK OFF)   8 OUNCES

EXTRA COMMENTS:
....

Dietary Journal

DIETARY	Vegetable	Protein	Carbohydrate	Fat	Dairy	Fruit	Calories
Breakfast							
Snack							
Lunch							
Snack							
Dinner							
Daily Food Totals							

DID YOU REACH YOUR DAILY DIETARY GOAL?   YES   NO   *IF NO, why?*   TIME   WORK   STRESS   HUNGRY   MOOD

DID YOU TAKE YOUR MULTIPLE VITAMIN?   YES   NO   OTHER SUPPLEMENTS ....

EAT OUT?   YES   NO   IF YES, GOOD OR BAD   CURRENT WEIGHT .... POUNDS.

WATER INTAKE (CHECK OFF)   8 OUNCES

EXTRA COMMENTS:
....

Dietary Journal

DIETARY	Vegetable	Protein	Carbohydrate	Fat	Dairy	Fruit	Calories
Breakfast							
Snack							
Lunch							
Snack							
Dinner							
Daily Food Totals							

DID YOU REACH YOUR DAILY DIETARY GOAL?   YES   NO   *IF NO, why?*   TIME   WORK   STRESS   HUNGRY   MOOD

DID YOU TAKE YOUR MULTIPLE VITAMIN?   YES   NO   OTHER SUPPLEMENTS ....

EAT OUT?   YES   NO   IF YES, GOOD OR BAD   CURRENT WEIGHT .... POUNDS.

WATER INTAKE (CHECK OFF)   8 OUNCES

EXTRA COMMENTS:
....

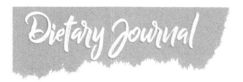

DAY 24

DIETARY	Vegetable	Protein	Carbohydrate	Fat	Dairy	Fruit	Calories
Breakfast							
Snack							
Lunch							
Snack							
Dinner							
Daily Food Totals							

DID YOU REACH YOUR DAILY DIETARY GOAL?   YES   NO   *IF NO, why?*   TIME   WORK   STRESS   HUNGRY   MOOD

DID YOU TAKE YOURMULTIPLE VITAMIN?   YES   NO   OTHER SUPPLEMENTS ....

EAT OUT?   YES   NO   IF YES, GOOD OR BAD   CURRENT WEIGHT .... POUNDS.

WATER INTAKE (CHECK OFF)   8 OUNCES

EXTRA COMMENTS:
....

Dietary Journal

DIETARY	Vegetable	Protein	Carbohydrate	Fat	Dairy	Fruit	Calories
Breakfast							
Snack							
Lunch							
Snack							
Dinner							
Daily Food Totals							

DID YOU REACH YOUR DAILY DIETARY GOAL?　　YES　　NO　*IF NO, why?*　　TIME　　WORK　　STRESS　　HUNGRY　　MOOD

DID YOU TAKE YOURMULTIPLE VITAMIN?　　YES　　NO　　OTHER SUPPLEMENTS ....

EAT OUT?　　YES　　NO　　IF YES, GOOD OR BAD　　CURRENT WEIGHT .... POUNDS.

WATER INTAKE (CHECK OFF)　　　　　　　　　8 OUNCES

EXTRA COMMENTS:
....

Dietary Journal

DAY 26

DIETARY	Vegetable	Protein	Carbohydrate	Fat	Dairy	Fruit	Calories
Breakfast							
Snack							
Lunch							
Snack							
Dinner							
Daily Food Totals							

DID YOU REACH YOUR DAILY DIETARY GOAL?   YES   NO   **IF NO, why?**   TIME   WORK   STRESS   HUNGRY   MOOD

DID YOU TAKE YOUR MULTIPLE VITAMIN?   YES   NO   OTHER SUPPLEMENTS ....

EAT OUT?   YES   NO   IF YES, GOOD OR BAD   CURRENT WEIGHT .... POUNDS.

WATER INTAKE (CHECK OFF)   8 OUNCES

EXTRA COMMENTS:
....

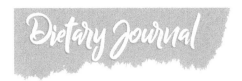

DIETARY	Vegetable	Protein	Carbohydrate	Fat	Dairy	Fruit	Calories
Breakfast							
Snack							
Lunch							
Snack							
Dinner							
Daily Food Totals							

DID YOU REACH YOUR DAILY DIETARY GOAL?   YES   NO *IF NO, why?*   TIME   WORK   STRESS   HUNGRY   MOOD

DID YOU TAKE YOURMULTIPLE VITAMIN?   YES   NO   OTHER SUPPLEMENTS ....

EAT OUT?   YES   NO   IF YES, GOOD OR BAD   CURRENT WEIGHT .... POUNDS.

WATER INTAKE (CHECK OFF)   8 OUNCES

EXTRA COMMENTS:
....

Dietary Journal

DAY 28

DIETARY	Vegetable	Protein	Carbohydrate	Fat	Dairy	Fruit	Calories
Breakfast							
Snack							
Lunch							
Snack							
Dinner							
Daily Food Totals							

DID YOU REACH YOUR DAILY DIETARY GOAL? YES NO *IF NO, why?* TIME WORK STRESS HUNGRY MOOD

DID YOU TAKE YOUR MULTIPLE VITAMIN? YES NO OTHER SUPPLEMENTS ....

EAT OUT? YES NO IF YES, GOOD OR BAD CURRENT WEIGHT .... POUNDS.

WATER INTAKE (CHECK OFF) 8 OUNCES

EXTRA COMMENTS:
....

66

Dietary Journal

DIETARY	Vegetable	Protein	Carbohydrate	Fat	Dairy	Fruit	Calories
Breakfast							
Snack							
Lunch							
Snack							
Dinner							
Daily Food Totals							

DID YOU REACH YOUR DAILY DIETARY GOAL?   YES   NO   *IF NO, why?*   TIME   WORK   STRESS   HUNGRY   MOOD

DID YOU TAKE YOURMULTIPLE VITAMIN?   YES   NO   OTHER SUPPLEMENTS ....

EAT OUT?   YES   NO   IF YES, GOOD OR BAD   CURRENT WEIGHT .... POUNDS.

WATER INTAKE (CHECK OFF)   8 OUNCES

EXTRA COMMENTS:
....

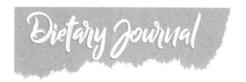

DAY 30

DIETARY	Vegetable	Protein	Carbohydrate	Fat	Dairy	Fruit	Calories
Breakfast							
Snack							
Lunch							
Snack							
Dinner							
Daily Food Totals							

DID YOU REACH YOUR DAILY DIETARY GOAL?   YES   NO   *IF NO, why?*   TIME   WORK   STRESS   HUNGRY   MOOD

DID YOU TAKE YOUR MULTIPLE VITAMIN?   YES   NO   OTHER SUPPLEMENTS ....

EAT OUT?   YES   NO   IF YES, GOOD OR BAD   CURRENT WEIGHT .... POUNDS.

WATER INTAKE (CHECK OFF)   8 OUNCES

EXTRA COMMENTS:
....

Daily Eating Healthy Intake & Habits

WEEK 1   CLICK OFF THE LIST FOR KEEPING ON TRACK

DAY	ALCOHOL YES/NO	PASTRIES, WHITE PRODUCTS	HIGH SUGARFOODS YES/NO	JUICE	1-2 GOOD FRUIT	2 SALADS	RESISTANCE WORKOUT AND/OR CARDIO(TIME)	2-3 VEGGIES, 1 COMPLEX CARB	3-4 LEAN PROTIEN	WATER - 8 8oz. GLASSES
1										
2										
3										
4										
5										
6										
7										

GOOD HABIT ☐ BAD HABIT, NEVER OR VERY LIMITED

Daily Eating Healthy Intake & Habits

WEEK 2　　　　CLICK OFF THE LIST FOR KEEPING ON TRACK

DAY	ALCOHOL YES/NO	PASTRIES, WHITE PRODUCTS	HIGH SUGARFOODS YES/NO	JUICE	1-2 GOOD FRUIT	2 SALADS	RESISTANCE WORKOUT AND/OR CARDIO(TIME)	2-3 VEGGIES, 1 COMPLEX CARB	3-4 LEAN PROTIEN	WATER - 8 8oz. GLASSES
1										
2										
3										
4										
5										
6										
7										

GOOD HABIT　　　BAD HABIT, NEVER OR VERY LIMITED

Daily Eating Healthy Intake & Habits

WEEK 3   CLICK OFF THE LIST FOR KEEPING ON TRACK

DAY	ALCOHOL YES/NO	PASTRIES, WHITE PRODUCTS	HIGH SUGARFOODS YES/NO	JUICE	1-2 GOOD FRUIT	2 SALADS	RESISTANCE WORKOUT AND/OR CARDIO(TIME)	2-3 VEGGIES, 1 COMPLEX CARB	3-4 LEAN PROTIEN	WATER - 8 8oz. GLASSES
1										
2										
3										
4										
5										
6										
7										

GOOD HABIT   BAD HABIT, NEVER OR VERY LIMITED

Daily Eating Healthy Intake & Habits

WEEK 4   CLICK OFF THE LIST FOR KEEPING ON TRACK

DAY	ALCOHOL YES/NO	PASTRIES, WHITE PRODUCTS	HIGH SUGARFOODS YES/NO	JUICE	1-2 GOOD FRUIT	2 SALADS	RESISTANCE WORKOUT AND/OR CARDIO(TIME)	2-3 VEGGIES, 1 COMPLEX CARB	3-4 LEAN PROTIEN	WATER - 8 8oz. GLASSES
1										
2										
3										
4										
5										
6										
7										

☐ GOOD HABIT   ☐ BAD HABIT, NEVER OR VERY LIMITED

YOUR 30 DAY TOTAL BODY TONE UP PLAN

BY DOUG BENNETT, TOP AMERICAN TRAINER

WEEKLY MEASUREMENTS:

PICK ONE DAY OF WEEK (SUGGEST SUNDAY OR MONDAY)

WEEK	BODY FAT %	WEIGHT (LBS.)	INCHES (BELLY)	INCHES (R. ARM)	INCHES (R. THIGH)
1					
2					
3					
4					

SHORT-TERM FITNESS GOAL: FIRST 30 DAYS...

SECOND 30 DAYS: ....

Weekly Schedule of Resistance Training

	Monday	Tuesday	Wednesday	Thursday	Friday	Saturaday	Sunday
WEEK 1							
WEEK 2							
WEEK 3							
WEEK 4							

Location Code:

Home	H
Gym	G
Travel	T

Body Code:

Back	B	Shoulders	SH
Legs	L	Chest	CH
Biceps	Bi	Abs	AB
Tricepts	Tri	Calves	CA

Example:

Week 1	B / Bi / AB / H
MONDAY	45 min

Bottom Line Quick Reference Food Guide

LEAN PROTEIN:
(Free Range, Organic)

- Turkey Breast
- Salmon
- Tofu
- Chicken breast (Low-Fat Organic)
- Cottage Cheese
- Seeds (Hemp, Flax)
- Lean Beef
- Organic Ground Beef, Chicken or Turkey
- White Tuna
- Egg Whites, Organic Eggs
- Shrimp
- White Fish
- Scallops
- Unsweetened Greek Yogurt
- Filet Mignin
- Organic Low-Fat Milk or Organic Unsweetend Non-Dairy Milk

LOW SPIKE SUGARS:
(Organic)

- Brown Rice (Short Grain)
- Black Beans
- Barley
- Wild Rice
- Yams
- Brown Rice Cakes
- Bulgur Wheat
- Sweet Potato
- Whole Oats (Organic)
- Lentil, KidneyBeans
- Bread
- Quinoa

GOOD FRUIT:
(Organic)

- Apples
- Apricots
- Blackberries
- Blueberries
- Boysenberries
- Cantaloupe
- Oranges
- Peaches
- Pears
- Pineapples
- Raspberries
- Strawberries
- Tangerines
- Nectarines
- Bananas(limited)
  *Slightly Green = less Sugar

GOOD VEGETABLES:
(Organic)
(1 Cup cooked or 1/2 Cup Raw = 1 Serving)

- Artichoke Hearts
- Asparagus
- Black Beans
- Broccoli
- Brussel Sprouts
- Cabbage
- Carrots
- Cauliflower
- Greens
- Leeks
- Okra
- Peppers (red or green)
- Spinach
- Sauerkraut
- Sprouts
- Tomato
- Zucchini
- Kale

Shopping list Essentials

PROTEIN:

- Chicken (Free Range, Organic: Ground, Breast or Bone-in)
- Turkey (Free Range, Organic: Ground, Breast or Bone-in)
- Fish
- Turkey Sausage
- Chicken Sausage
- Turkey Bacon
- Firm Tofu
- Flank Steak, Organic Beef (Ground, 93% lean), Filet, Sirloin (Lean Cuts)
- Crab
- Canned White or Tune (1x week)
- Egg White or Egg
- Shrimp
- All Natural/Low Sodium Deli Turkey (Limited)
- Protein Powders: Hemp, Pea protein, Brown rice protein, Egg protein and/or Organic whey protein powder
- Lentils, Legumes
- Raw Nut Butters

VEGETABLES & HERBS:

- Kale
- Asparagus
- Broccoli
- Cabbage
- Carrots
- Salad Greens
- Spinach
- Tomato
- Zucchini
- Cauliflower
- Celery
- Sweet Potato
- Avocado
- Pappers
- Mushrooms
- Cliantro
- basil
- Rosemary
- Garlic

DAIRY:
Organic, Low-Fat

- Cottage Cheese
  (Low-Fat, No Preservatives)
- Yogurt (Plain Greek: Add Freash Fruit and/or Raw Nuts)
- Fresh Parmesan Cheese
  (No Cellulose)
- Feta (Little For Taste)
- Organic Low-Fat Milk Or Butter

FRUITS:
Organic Fresh or Frozen (Cheaper)

- Apples
- Blueberries
- Strawberries
- Oranges
- Pears
- Raspberries
- Peaches
- Banana
- Water Melon

Shopping list Essentials

(Continued)

Beverages:

- [ ] Natural Seltzer Water
- [ ] Organic Low-Fat Milk, Unsweetened Organic Non-dairy Coconut or Almond Milk
- [ ] Skim milk
- [ ] Nonfat/Low Fat Soy Milk
- [ ] Decaf Coffee
- [ ] Herbal Teas

Cereals:

- [ ] Bran Flakes (Health Valley)
- [ ] Whole Oats(McCann's, Country Choice)
- [ ] Oat Bran
- [ ] Ezekiel Brand

Bread, Crackers & Starches:

- [ ] Ezekiel Brand Bread
- [ ] Wasa Crackers
- [ ] Whole Crain Crackers
- [ ] Sourdough/whole Grain Pretzels
- [ ] Brown Rice Cakes (Lundberg Brand)
- [ ] Whole Grain Pasta (Brown rice, Quinoa)
- [ ] Whole Grain Tortillas (Flax, Quinoa, Brown Rice)
- [ ] Whole Grain Pita
- [ ] Short Grain Pita, Short Grain Brown Rice
- [ ] Quinoa
- [ ] Steel Cut Oats(Organic Only)
- [ ] Organic Corn Tortilla Chips
- [ ] Wild Rice
- [ ] Black Beans
- [ ] Lentils

Fats:

- [ ] 100% Canola Oil & Spray (Spectrum)
- [ ] Buttery Spread (Earth Balance Only)
- [ ] Mayonnaise (Spectrum)
- [ ] Raw Almonds, Cashews & Or peanuts
- [ ] Almond or Natual Peanut Butter
- [ ] Flax Seeds, Hemp Seeds
- [ ] Avocado
- [ ] Organic Nut & Dried Fruit Mix

AFTERWORD

Well that's it for the TOTAL BODY WORKOUT GUIDE. I hope you will try your best and stick to the program as closely as possible. The key to losing weight and great results is making mindful food choices and training with intensity based upon your fitness level. Always try to live by the rule of, "You are what you eat!". If you eat health, you'll be healthy. Simple, as that. Of course, exercise is a key component, but nutrition is the main factor to looking fit and faster results.

By the way, if you have any questions or concerns related to this or any of your fitness concerns. Please email me, Doug Bennett, at bsstudio@comcast.net Title the subject line, "30 DAY TOTAL BODY GUIDE".

Don't Forget to check out our Social Sites for FREE VIDEOS, TIPS and RECIPES:

Blog: www.fitactions.com

Instagram: www.instagram.com/FITACTIONS OR www.instagram.com/boxtobefit

Facebook: www.facebook.com/gogirlfit

YouTube: The Bennett Method https://www.youtube.com/user/fitgy321

SIGN UP FOR FREE WORKOUTS: CLICK HERE

Other Books and Programs:

Amazon:

The 6 Week Lower Body Fix: Your Ultimate Workout Plan To Help Get The Ultimate Legs, Bum & Body for Women.

The 6 Week Upper Body Fix: Your Ultimate 2-Phase Upper Body Workout Plan to Give You a Tone, Strong Upper Body, Flat Abs and Look Amazing - Fast!

Apple IApps:

Fitgirl Pro

15 Minute Metabolic Burners

Made in the USA
Las Vegas, NV
21 February 2024

86071193R00046